THE

GOUT

COOKBOOK

SARAH JACK

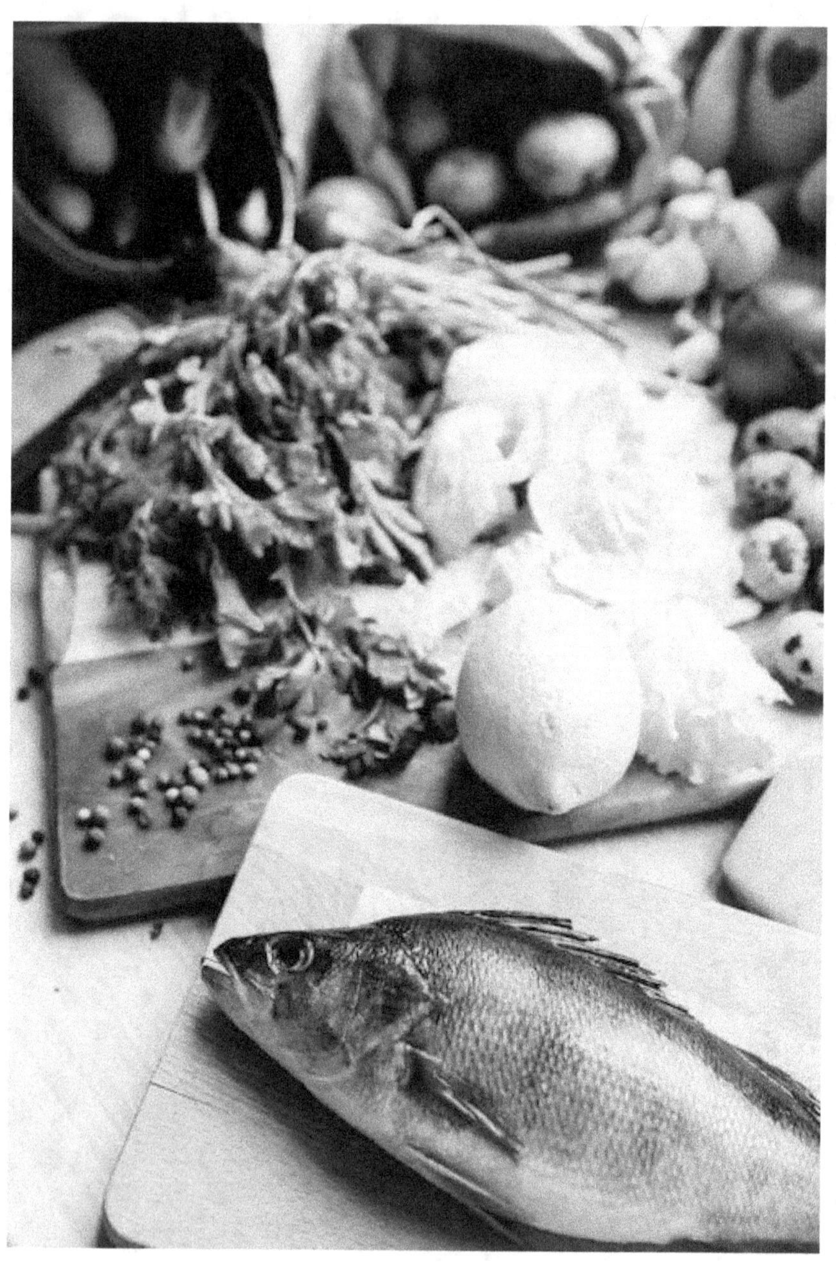

COPYRIGHT

TABLE OF CONTENTS

Table of Contents

COPYRIGHT 3

TABLE OF CONTENTS 4

INTRODUCTION 6

IMPORATNCE OF DIET FOR MANAGING GOUT
.... 11

ESSENTIAL FOODS FOR MANAGING GOUT . 15

PRACTICAL TIPS FOR INCORPORATING GOUT-
FRIENDLY FOODS INTO YOUR LIFESTYLE .. 19

GOUT DIET RECIPES 23

INTRODUCTION

GOUT

Gout, an age-old ailment once dubbed the "disease of kings," has endured across time, impacting individuals regardless of their societal standing. This variant of inflammatory arthritis, marked by sudden and agonizing discomfort, swelling, and inflammation in the joints, notably the big toe, has intrigued medical practitioners for generations. Delvee into the complexities of gout, ranging from its fundamental causes to its methods of management and prevention.

- **Understanding the Fundamentals of Gout**

The primary cause of gout lies in the accumulation of uric acid crystals within the joints, inducing inflammation and discomfort. Uric acid, a byproduct of purine metabolism, typically exits the body through urine. However, in individuals with hyperuricemia, where uric acid levels in the bloodstream are elevated, these crystals can form and deposit in the joints, provoking gout attacks. While the big toe often bears the brunt, gout can also affect various other joints such as the ankles, knees, wrists, and fingers.

- **Contributing Factors to Gout Development**

Numerous elements contribute to the onset of gout. Genetics play a substantial role, with certain individuals inheriting a predisposition to hyperuricemia. Additionally, dietary patterns abundant in purine-rich foods like red meat, shellfish, and alcohol can heighten uric acid levels, escalating the risk of gout. Obesity, specific medical conditions such as kidney disease, and the use of medications like diuretics can further exacerbate the propensity for gout episodes.

- **Indicators and Symptoms**

Gout episodes typically manifest abruptly, frequently striking during nighttime hours. The afflicted joint swells, becomes tender to the touch, and experiences intense pain, rendering even minor movements unbearable. Inflammation often causes the area to appear red and feel warm. The duration of gout attacks varies, ranging from several days to weeks. In persistent cases, recurrent gout episodes can lead to joint impairment and deformities.

- **Diagnosis and Treatment Approaches**

Diagnosing gout typically involves a blend of clinical evaluation, medical history assessment, and laboratory examinations. Imaging techniques such as X-rays or ultrasound may also be employed to assess joint integrity. Once diagnosed, the treatment of gout aims to assuage pain and inflammation during acute episodes and forestall future occurrences. Nonsteroidal anti-inflammatory drugs (NSAIDs), corticosteroids, and colchicine are frequently prescribed to manage acute symptoms. Long-term management entails medications like allopurinol or febuxostat to diminish uric acid levels in the bloodstream and deter crystal formation.

- **Lifestyle Adjustments and Prevention Strategies**

Lifestyle modifications play a pivotal role in gout management. Sustaining a healthy body weight, embracing a balanced diet low in purine-rich foods, moderating alcohol intake, and ensuring adequate hydration can all contribute to reducing the frequency and severity of gout attacks. Moreover, regular physical activity can enhance joint functionality and overall well-being, aiding in gout prevention.

- **Conclusion**

Gout, a multifaceted form of arthritis, presents significant hurdles for those grappling with its incapacitating symptoms. Nevertheless, with a comprehensive understanding of its origins, manifestations, and therapeutic avenues, individuals can effectively navigate the challenges posed by gout and enhance their quality of life. By adopting lifestyle adjustments and proactive prevention measures, individuals can mitigate the impact of gout on their health and vitality, fostering a future free from pain and discomfort.

IMPORATNCE OF DIET FOR MANAGING GOUT

The role of diet in managing gout is pivotal, given that certain food choices can either contribute to the initiation of gout attacks or assist in alleviating symptoms and preventing future flare-ups. Recognizing how diet impacts gout and making suitable dietary adjustments can notably enhance the management of this condition. Here's why diet holds significance in the management of gout:

Purine Content: Purines, substances present in various foods, undergo metabolism into uric acid within the body. Elevated levels of uric acid can precipitate gout attacks. Foods abundant in purines, such as red meat, organ meats (like liver and kidney), shellfish, and specific fish varieties (like anchovies and sardines), can elevate uric acid levels and instigate gout flare-ups. Hence, limiting the consumption of these purine-rich foods is imperative for effectively managing gout.

Alcohol Consumption: The consumption of alcohol, especially beer and spirits, is strongly linked to an augmented risk of gout attacks. Alcohol intake can both elevate uric acid levels and impede the body's capacity to expel uric acid, rendering individuals more susceptible to gout. Moderating or abstaining from alcohol, particularly beer and spirits, can aid in diminishing the frequency and severity of gout attacks.

Weight Management: Obesity represents a notable risk factor for gout, given its association with heightened uric acid levels. Embracing a nutritious diet and maintaining a healthy weight can assist in lowering uric acid levels and reducing the propensity for gout attacks. A well-rounded diet comprising fruits, vegetables, whole grains, and lean proteins can facilitate weight management and foster overall health.

Hydration: Adequate hydration is indispensable for gout management, as it helps deter the formation of uric acid crystals in the joints. Consuming ample water and other nonalcoholic beverages aids in diluting uric acid in the bloodstream and facilitating its elimination via urine. Sufficient hydration also aids in flushing out toxins, thereby diminishing the likelihood of gout attacks.

Anti-Inflammatory Foods: Certain foods possess anti-inflammatory properties, which can assuage gout symptoms. Antioxidant-rich foods like cherries, berries, and dark leafy greens have demonstrated efficacy in reducing inflammation and lowering uric acid levels. Integrating these anti-inflammatory foods into the diet can complement medical intervention and provide relief from gout symptoms.

Dietary Supplements: Some dietary supplements, such as vitamin C and fish oil, may confer benefits in managing gout. Vitamin C supplements have been shown to decrease uric acid levels, while fish oil supplements exhibit anti-inflammatory properties that can mitigate gout-related inflammation. Nevertheless, consulting with a healthcare professional prior to initiating any dietary supplements is essential, particularly for individuals with other medical conditions or those taking medications.

In summary, diet plays a pivotal role in managing gout by influencing uric acid levels, inflammation, and overall well-being. Implementing dietary modifications, such as curtailing the consumption of purine-rich foods, moderating alcohol intake, maintaining a healthy weight, staying adequately hydrated, and incorporating anti-inflammatory foods, can aid in preventing gout attacks and enhancing the quality of life for individuals grappling with this condition. Collaborating closely with healthcare professionals, including dietitians or nutritionists, is crucial for devising a tailored diet plan that aligns with individual needs and supports gout management objectives.

ESSENTIAL FOODS FOR MANAGING GOUT

Managing gout through diet involves incorporating foods that can help lower uric acid levels, reduce inflammation, and promote overall joint health. While avoiding purine-rich foods and alcohol is essential, there are several foods that individuals with gout can include in their diet to help manage symptoms and prevent flare-ups. Here are some essential foods for managing gout:

Cherries: Cherries, particularly tart cherries, are rich in antioxidants called anthocyanins, which have anti-inflammatory properties. Consuming cherries or cherry juice has been associated with a reduced risk of gout attacks and lower serum uric acid levels. Adding cherries to your diet regularly may help alleviate gout symptoms and prevent flare-ups.

Berries: Berries such as strawberries, blueberries, and raspberries are packed with antioxidants and vitamin C, which have anti-inflammatory properties. Including berries in your diet can help reduce inflammation associated with gout and provide relief from symptoms.

Dark Leafy Greens: Dark leafy greens like spinach, kale, and Swiss chard are low in purines and rich in vitamins, minerals, and antioxidants. These greens can help alkalize the body and reduce inflammation, making them beneficial for individuals with gout. Incorporating dark leafy greens into salads, smoothies, or cooked dishes can support gout management.

Whole Grains: Whole grains like oats, quinoa, barley, and brown rice are high in fiber and low in purines, making them suitable choices for individuals with gout. Fiber-rich foods can help regulate blood sugar levels and promote satiety, which may aid in weight management—an important aspect of gout management.

Nuts and Seeds: Nuts and seeds, such as almonds, walnuts, flaxseeds, and chia seeds, are rich in healthy fats, fiber, and plant-based protein. They can be included in the diet as snacks or added to salads, yogurt, or smoothies. Nuts and seeds provide essential nutrients and may help reduce inflammation associated with gout.

Fatty Fish: Fatty fish like salmon, mackerel, trout, and sardines are rich in omega-3 fatty acids, which have anti-inflammatory properties. Consuming fatty fish regularly can help reduce inflammation in the body and may lower the risk of gout attacks. Grilling, baking, or broiling fish is recommended to retain its nutritional benefits.

Low-Fat Dairy Products: Low-fat dairy products such as yogurt, milk, and cheese are excellent sources of calcium and protein. Studies have shown that consuming low-fat dairy products may help lower uric acid levels and reduce the risk of gout attacks. Opting for low-fat or non-fat dairy options can provide essential nutrients without the added saturated fats.

Water: Staying hydrated is essential for managing gout, as it helps flush out uric acid from the body through urine. Drinking plenty of water throughout the day can help prevent uric acid crystal formation and reduce the risk of gout attacks. Aim to drink at least 8-10 glasses of water daily, and consider increasing your intake during hot weather or physical activity.

Incorporating these essential foods into your diet can help support gout management and reduce the frequency and severity of gout attacks. However, it's essential to maintain a balanced diet overall, rich in fruits, vegetables, whole grains, lean proteins, and healthy fats, while limiting purine-rich foods and alcohol intake.

PRACTICAL TIPS FOR INCORPORATING GOUT-FRIENDLY FOODS INTO YOUR LIFESTYLE

Incorporating gout-friendly foods into your lifestyle can be a key aspect of managing this condition effectively. Here are some practical tips to help you integrate these foods into your daily routine:

Plan Your Meals: Take some time to plan your meals for the week ahead. Include a variety of gout-friendly foods such as fruits, vegetables, whole grains, and lean proteins in your meal plans.

Focus on Fruits and Vegetables: Aim to make fruits and vegetables the mainstay of your meals. Incorporate a colorful variety of fruits and vegetables into your dishes to ensure you get a wide range of nutrients and antioxidants.

Experiment with Recipes: Look for recipes that feature gout-friendly ingredients and experiment with new dishes. Try incorporating more plant-based meals into your diet, such as salads, stir-fries, and vegetable-based soups.

Choose Whole Grains: Opt for whole grains such as brown rice, quinoa, oats, and barley instead of refined grains. Whole grains are rich in fiber and nutrients and can help promote satiety and regulate blood sugar levels.

Include Lean Proteins: Choose lean sources of protein such as poultry, fish, tofu, and legumes. These protein sources are lower in purines compared to red meat and organ meats, making them a better choice for individuals with gout.

Snack Smart: Keep gout-friendly snacks on hand for when hunger strikes between meals. Choose snacks like fresh fruits, raw vegetables with hummus, nuts, or Greek yogurt to satisfy your cravings without exacerbating gout symptoms.

Stay Hydrated: Drink plenty of water throughout the day to help flush out uric acid from your body and prevent gout attacks. Carry a water bottle with you wherever you go to ensure you stay hydrated.

Limit Alcohol: If you choose to drink alcohol, do so in moderation and opt for gout-friendly options like wine or beer in small quantities. Avoid excessive consumption of beer and spirits, which are high in purines and can trigger gout attacks.

Read Labels: When shopping for packaged foods, read the labels carefully to check for ingredients that may exacerbate gout symptoms. Avoid foods high in purines, added sugars, and unhealthy fats.

Seek Support: Joining a support group or connecting with others who have gout can provide valuable tips, encouragement, and motivation on incorporating gout-friendly foods into your lifestyle. Share recipes, meal ideas, and success stories with fellow gout sufferers to stay inspired on your journey to better health.

By following these practical tips and making gradual changes to your eating habits, you can successfully incorporate gout-friendly foods into your lifestyle and better manage this condition over the long term. Remember to consult with your healthcare provider or a registered dietitian for personalized advice and guidance tailored to your specific needs and preferences.

GOUT DIET RECIPES

Miso-Glazed Eggplant with Quinoa and Edamame

Ingredients:

- 1 large eggplant, sliced into 1/2-inch rounds

- 2 tablespoons olive oil

- 1/4 cup white miso paste

- 2 tablespoons mirin (sweet rice wine)

- 1 tablespoon rice vinegar

- 1 clove garlic, minced

- 1 cup cooked quinoa

- 1 cup shelled edamame, cooked

- 1 scallion, thinly sliced (optional)

- Sesame seeds for garnish (optional)

Instructions:

- Preheat oven to 400°F (200°C). Brush eggplant slices with olive oil and bake for 15-20 minutes, flipping halfway through, until tender.

- Meanwhile, whisk together miso paste, mirin, rice vinegar, and garlic in a small bowl.

- In a pan, heat a tablespoon of olive oil. Add cooked quinoa and edamame, and stir-fry for a few minutes.

- To assemble, place baked eggplant slices on a plate. Top with the quinoa-edamame mixture and drizzle with miso glaze.

- Garnish with sliced scallions and sesame seeds (optional).

Spiced Lentil and Butternut Squash Stew

Ingredients:

- 1 tablespoon olive oil

- 1 onion, chopped

- 2 carrots, chopped

- 1 celery stalk, chopped

- 2 cloves garlic, minced

- 1 teaspoon ground cumin

- 1/2 teaspoon turmeric

- 1/4 teaspoon ground coriander

- 1 (14.5 oz) can diced tomatoes, undrained

- 4 cups vegetable broth

- 1 cup brown lentils, rinsed

- 1 butternut squash, peeled and chopped

- 1 cup chopped kale or spinach

- Salt and pepper to taste

Instructions:

- Heat olive oil in a large pot over medium heat. Add onion, carrots, and celery, and cook until softened, about 5 minutes.

- Stir in garlic, cumin, turmeric, and coriander. Cook for an additional minute.

- Add diced tomatoes, vegetable broth, lentils, and butternut squash. Bring to a boil, then reduce heat and simmer for 30 minutes, or until lentils and squash are tender.

- Stir in kale or spinach and cook until wilted.

- Season with salt and pepper to taste.

Watercress and Fennel Soup with Toasted Walnuts

Ingredients:

- 1 tablespoon olive oil

- 1 onion, chopped

- 1 fennel bulb, chopped

- 2 cloves garlic, minced

- 4 cups vegetable broth

- 2 cups chopped watercress

- 1/2 cup chopped walnuts, toasted

- Salt and pepper to taste

Instructions:

- Heat olive oil in a large pot over medium heat. Add onion and fennel, and cook until softened, about 5 minutes.

- Stir in garlic and cook for an additional minute.

- Add vegetable broth and bring to a boil. Reduce heat and simmer for 10 minutes.

- Stir in watercress and cook for 2-3 minutes, or until wilted.

- Using an immersion blender or in batches, puree the soup until smooth. Season with salt and pepper to taste.

- Ladle soup into bowls and top with toasted walnuts.

Amaranth Porridge with Roasted Pears and Pecans

Ingredients:

- 1/2 cup amaranth, rinsed

- 1 1/2 cups milk (dairy or non-dairy)

- 1/4 cup water

- 1/4 teaspoon ground cinnamon

- 2 ripe pears, halved and cored

- 1 tablespoon olive oil

- 1/4 cup chopped pecans

- Maple syrup or honey (optional)

Instructions:

- In a saucepan, combine amaranth, milk, water, and cinnamon. Bring to a boil, then reduce heat and simmer for 20-25 minutes, or until amaranth is cooked through and porridge thickens.

- Meanwhile, preheat oven to 400°F (200°C). Toss pear halves with olive oil and place cut side down on a baking sheet. Roast for 15-20 minutes, or until tender.

- Serve amaranth porridge topped with roasted pears, chopped pecans, and a drizzle of maple syrup or honey (optional).

Coconut Curry Mussels with Mango Salsa

Ingredients:

- 1 pound mussels, debearded and rinsed

- 1 tablespoon olive oil

- 1 onion, chopped

- 2 cloves garlic, minced

- 1 tablespoon curry powder

- 1 teaspoon ground ginger

- 1 (14.5 oz) can coconut milk

- 1 cup vegetable broth

- 1/2 cup chopped red bell pepper

- 1/4 cup chopped green beans

- 1 mango, diced

- 1/4 cup chopped red onion

- 1 tablespoon lime juice

- 1/4 cup chopped fresh cilantro

- Salt and pepper to taste

Instructions:

- In a large pot, heat olive oil over medium heat. Add onion and garlic, and cook until softened, about 5 minutes.

- Stir in curry powder and ginger. Cook for an additional minute.

- Add coconut milk, vegetable broth, red bell pepper, and green beans. Bring to a simmer.

- Add mussels to the pot and cover. Cook for 5-7 minutes, or until mussels open. Discard any unopened mussels.

- While mussels cook, combine diced mango, red onion, lime juice, and cilantro in a small bowl.

- Serve mussels in the coconut curry sauce with mango salsa on the side.

Buckwheat Pancakes with Berries and Chia Seed Jam

Ingredients:

- 1 cup buckwheat flour

- 1/2 cup milk (dairy or non-dairy)

- 1 egg, beaten

- 1 tablespoon melted coconut oil

- 1/2 teaspoon baking powder

- 1/4 teaspoon salt

- 1 cup mixed berries

- 1/4 cup chia seeds

- 1/4 cup water

- 1 tablespoon maple syrup (optional)

Instructions:

- In a bowl, whisk together buckwheat flour, milk, egg, melted coconut oil, baking powder, and salt.

- Heat a lightly oiled pan over medium heat. Pour batter into small circles to form pancakes.

- Cook for 2-3 minutes per side, or until golden brown.

- While pancakes cook, combine berries, chia seeds, water, and maple syrup (optional) in a small saucepan. Heat over low heat until berries soften and mixture thickens.

- Serve pancakes topped with chia seed jam and additional berries.

Sprouted Mung Bean Salad with Tahini Dressing

Ingredients:

- 1 cup sprouted mung beans, rinsed and drained

- 1 cup chopped cucumber

- 1/2 cup chopped cherry tomatoes

- 1/4 cup chopped red onion

- 1/4 cup chopped fresh parsley

For the Tahini Dressing:

- 1/4 cup tahini

- 2 tablespoons lemon juice

- 1 tablespoon olive oil

- 1 clove garlic, minced

- 1/4 cup water

- Salt and pepper to taste

Instructions:

- In a large bowl, combine sprouted mung beans, cucumber, tomatoes, red onion, and parsley.

- To make the tahini dressing, whisk together tahini, lemon juice, olive oil, garlic, water, salt, and pepper in a small bowl until smooth.

- Pour the dressing over the salad and toss to coat. Serve chilled.

Quinoa Tabouli with Grilled Halloumi

Ingredients:

- 1 cup quinoa, rinsed

- 1 1/2 cups boiling water

- 1 cup chopped cucumber

- 1 cup chopped cherry tomatoes

- 1/2 cup chopped fresh parsley

- 1/4 cup chopped fresh mint

- 2 tablespoons olive oil

- 1 tablespoon lemon juice

- 1/4 teaspoon salt

- 8 ounces halloumi cheese, sliced

- Olive oil for grilling (optional)

Instructions:

- In a saucepan, combine quinoa and boiling water. Bring to a boil, then reduce heat and simmer for 15 minutes, or until quinoa is cooked through and fluffy. Set aside to cool.

- In a large bowl, combine cooled quinoa, cucumber, tomatoes, parsley, and mint.

- In a separate bowl, whisk together olive oil, lemon juice, and salt.

- Pour the dressing over the quinoa mixture and toss to coat.

- Heat a grill pan or grill over medium heat. Brush halloumi slices with olive oil (optional). Grill for 2-3 minutes per side, or until golden brown and slightly crispy.

- Serve tabbouleh salad with grilled halloumi cheese.

Roasted Chickpea and Butternut Squash Salad with Lemon Vinaigrette

Ingredients:

- 1 butternut squash, peeled and chopped

- 1 tablespoon olive oil

- 1 (15 oz) can chickpeas, drained and rinsed

- 1/2 cup chopped red onion

- 1/4 cup crumbled feta cheese (optional)

- 1/4 cup chopped fresh parsley

For the Lemon Vinaigrette:

- 2 tablespoons olive oil

- 1 tablespoon lemon juice

- 1 teaspoon Dijon mustard

- 1/2 teaspoon honey

- Salt and pepper to taste

Instructions:

- Preheat oven to 400°F (200°C). Toss butternut squash with olive oil and spread on a baking sheet. Roast for 20-25 minutes, or until tender.

- While squash roasts, heat a skillet over medium heat. Add chickpeas and cook for 5-7 minutes, or until slightly crispy.

- In a large bowl, combine roasted squash, chickpeas, red onion, feta cheese (optional), and parsley.

- To make the vinaigrette, whisk together olive oil, lemon juice, Dijon mustard, honey, salt, and pepper in a small bowl.

- Pour the vinaigrette over the salad and toss to coat. Serve chilled or at room temperature.

Salmon with Mango Salsa and Coconut Quinoa

Ingredients:

- 2 salmon fillets

- 1 tablespoon olive oil

- Salt and pepper to taste

- 1 cup cooked quinoa

- 1/2 cup chopped mango

- 1/4 cup chopped red onion

- 1/4 cup chopped fresh cilantro

- 1 tablespoon lime juice

- 1/4 cup unsweetened coconut flakes (toasted, optional)

Instructions:

- Preheat oven to 400°F (200°C). Season salmon fillets with olive oil, salt, and pepper. Place on a baking sheet lined with parchment paper.

- Bake for 15-20 minutes, or until cooked through.

- While salmon cooks, combine cooked quinoa, chopped mango, red onion, cilantro, and lime juice in a bowl.

- Toast coconut flakes in a dry skillet over medium heat for a few minutes, until golden brown (optional).

- Serve salmon over coconut quinoa (if using) and top with mango salsa.

Turkey Kefta Bowls with Roasted Vegetables and Tahini Sauce

Ingredients:

- 1 pound ground turkey

- 1/2 cup chopped onion

- 1/4 cup chopped fresh parsley

- 1 teaspoon ground cumin

- 1/2 teaspoon ground coriander

- Salt and pepper to taste

- 2 medium zucchini, chopped

- 1 red bell pepper, chopped

- 1 tablespoon olive oil

For the Tahini Sauce:

- 1/4 cup tahini

- 2 tablespoons lemon juice

- 1 tablespoon olive oil

- 1 clove garlic, minced

- 1/4 cup water

- Salt and pepper to taste

Instructions:

- Preheat oven to 400°F (200°C). In a large bowl, combine ground turkey, onion, parsley, cumin, coriander, salt, and pepper. Mix well.

- Form the mixture into small meatballs. Place meatballs on a baking sheet lined with parchment paper.

- Toss chopped zucchini and red bell pepper with olive oil and spread around the meatballs on the baking sheet.

- Bake for 20-25 minutes, or until meatballs are cooked through and vegetables are tender.

- To make the tahini sauce, whisk together tahini, lemon juice, olive oil, garlic, water, salt, and pepper in a small bowl until smooth.

- Serve turkey kefta bowls with roasted vegetables and drizzle with tahini sauce.

Spicy Black Bean Burgers with Sweet Potato Fries

Ingredients:

- 1 (15 oz) can black beans, rinsed and drained

- 1/2 cup cooked brown rice

- 1/4 cup chopped red onion

- 1 jalapeno pepper, seeded and minced (adjust for desired spice level)

- 1/4 cup chopped fresh cilantro

- 1 tablespoon olive oil

- 1 tablespoon lime juice

- 1 teaspoon ground cumin

- 1/2 teaspoon chili powder

- Salt and pepper to taste

- For the Sweet Potato Fries:

- 2 medium sweet potatoes, cut into wedges

- 1 tablespoon olive oil

- 1/2 teaspoon paprika

- Salt and pepper to taste

Instructions:

- In a large bowl, mash together black beans and cooked brown rice using a fork or potato masher. Don't mash completely - leave some texture.

- Stir in red onion, jalapeno pepper (optional), cilantro, olive oil, lime juice, cumin, chili powder, salt, and pepper.

- Form the mixture into patties. Heat a skillet over medium heat with a tablespoon of olive oil.

- Cook burgers for 4-5 minutes per side, or until golden brown and heated through.

- Preheat oven to 400°F (200°C). Toss sweet potato wedges with olive oil, paprika, salt, and pepper.

- Spread sweet potato wedges on a baking sheet lined with parchment paper. Bake for 20-25 minutes, or until tender and slightly crispy.

- Serve black bean burgers with sweet potato fries.

Shrimp Scampi with Zucchini Noodles

Ingredients:

- 1 pound shrimp, peeled and deveined

- 1 tablespoon olive oil

- 2 cloves garlic, minced

- 1/4 cup chopped red onion

- 1/2 cup dry white wine

- 1/4 cup chopped fresh parsley

- 1 tablespoon lemon juice

- 1/2 teaspoon red pepper flakes (optional)

- Salt and pepper to taste

- 2 medium zucchini, spiralized into noodles

Instructions:

- Heat olive oil in a large skillet over medium heat. Add shrimp and cook for 2-3 minutes per side, or until pink and cooked through. Remove shrimp from the pan and set aside.

- Add garlic and red onion to the pan and cook for a minute, until softened.

- Deglaze the pan with white wine, scraping up any browned bits. Let the wine simmer for a few minutes to reduce slightly.

- Stir in chopped parsley, lemon juice, red pepper flakes (optional), salt, and pepper.

- Add zucchini noodles to the pan and cook for 1-2 minutes, or until slightly softened.

- Return shrimp to the pan and toss to coat in the sauce. Serve immediately.

Rainbow Veggie Buddha Bowl with Turmeric Tahini Dressing

Ingredients:

- 1 cup cooked quinoa or brown rice

- 1/2 cup roasted chickpeas (seasoned with olive oil, salt, and pepper)

- 1 cup roasted vegetables (mix of broccoli florets, cauliflower florets, bell peppers)

- 1/2 cup chopped cucumber

- 1/4 cup shredded carrots

- 1/4 cup cherry tomatoes

- 1/4 cup crumbled feta cheese (optional)

For the Turmeric Tahini Dressing:

- 1/4 cup tahini

- 2 tablespoons lemon juice

- 1 tablespoon olive oil

- 1 clove garlic, minced

- 1/4 cup water

- 1/2 teaspoon ground turmeric

- Salt and pepper to taste

Instructions:

- Preheat oven to 400°F (200°C). Toss vegetables with olive oil, salt, and pepper. Roast for 20-25 minutes, or until tender-crisp.

- Prepare cooked quinoa or brown rice according to package instructions.

- To make the dressing, whisk together tahini, lemon juice, olive oil, garlic, water, turmeric, salt, and pepper in a small bowl until smooth.

- Assemble bowls with cooked quinoa or brown rice, roasted vegetables, roasted chickpeas, cucumber, carrots, cherry tomatoes, and crumbled feta cheese (optional).

- Drizzle with turmeric tahini dressing and serve.

Chicken and Vegetable Stir-Fry with Brown Rice Noodles

Ingredients:

- 1 pound boneless, skinless chicken breasts, sliced thin

- 1 tablespoon cornstarch

- 2 tablespoons soy sauce (low-sodium)

- 1 tablespoon rice vinegar

- 1 tablespoon sesame oil

- 1 tablespoon olive oil

- 1 red bell pepper, sliced

- 1 green bell pepper, sliced

- 1 cup broccoli florets

- 1/2 cup snow peas

- 1/4 cup chopped green onions

- 8 oz brown rice noodles, cooked according to package instructions

Instructions:

- In a bowl, toss chicken with cornstarch, soy sauce, rice vinegar, and sesame oil.

- Heat olive oil in a large skillet or wok over medium-high heat. Add chicken and cook for 5-7 minutes, or until cooked through. Remove chicken from the pan and set aside.

- Add bell peppers, broccoli florets, and snow peas to the pan. Stir-fry for 3-4 minutes, or until vegetables are tender-crisp.

- Return chicken to the pan and stir in green onions. Cook for an additional minute to heat through.

- Serve stir-fry over cooked brown rice noodles.

Salmon with Mango Avocado Salsa and Coconut Rice

Ingredients:

- 2 salmon fillets

- 1 tablespoon olive oil

- Salt and pepper to taste

- 1 cup cooked brown rice

- 1/2 cup chopped mango

- 1/2 cup chopped avocado

- 1/4 cup chopped red onion

- 1 tablespoon lime juice

- 1/4 cup chopped fresh cilantro

- 1/4 cup unsweetened coconut flakes (toasted, optional)

Instructions:

- Preheat oven to 400°F (200°C). Season salmon fillets with olive oil, salt, and pepper. Place on a baking sheet lined with parchment paper.

- Bake for 15-20 minutes, or until cooked through.

- While salmon cooks, prepare the salsa by combining chopped mango, avocado, red onion, lime juice, and cilantro in a bowl.

- Toast coconut flakes in a dry skillet over medium heat for a few minutes, until golden brown (optional).

- To make the coconut rice (optional), simply cook brown rice according to package instructions and stir in a few tablespoons of unsweetened coconut milk for a subtle flavor twist.

- Serve salmon over coconut rice (optional) and top with mango avocado salsa.

Gazpacho with Grilled Shrimp and Toasted Toasts

Ingredients:

- 4 ripe tomatoes, chopped

- 1 red bell pepper, chopped

- 1 cucumber, peeled and chopped

- 1/2 red onion, chopped

- 2 cloves garlic, minced

- 1/4 cup olive oil

- 2 tablespoons red wine vinegar

- 1 tablespoon lemon juice

- Salt and pepper to taste

For the Grilled Shrimp:

- 1 pound medium shrimp, peeled and deveined

- 1 tablespoon olive oil

- 1/2 teaspoon paprika

- Salt and pepper to taste

- For the Toasted Toasts:

- Slices of whole-wheat bread

Instructions:

- In a blender, combine chopped tomatoes, bell pepper, cucumber, red onion, garlic, olive oil, red wine vinegar, lemon juice, salt, and pepper. Blend until smooth.

- Chill gazpacho in the refrigerator for at least 1 hour.

- Preheat grill or grill pan to medium heat. Toss shrimp with olive oil, paprika, salt, and pepper.

- Grill shrimp for 2-3 minutes per side, or until pink and cooked through.

- Toast whole-wheat bread slices.

- Serve chilled gazpacho topped with grilled shrimp and a drizzle of olive oil (optional). Enjoy with toasted bread slices.

Turkey Meatloaf with Roasted Vegetables

Ingredients:

- 1 pound ground turkey

- 1/2 cup chopped onion

- 1/4 cup chopped bell pepper (any color)

- 1/4 cup chopped mushrooms

- 1/4 cup rolled oats

- 1 egg, beaten

- 1 tablespoon Worcestershire sauce

- 1 teaspoon dried thyme

- Salt and pepper to taste

For the Roasted Vegetables:

- 2 medium carrots, chopped

- 2 celery stalks, chopped

- 1 red onion, chopped

- 1 tablespoon olive oil

- Salt and pepper to taste

Instructions:

- Preheat oven to 375°F (190°C). In a large bowl, combine ground turkey, onion, bell pepper, mushrooms, rolled oats, egg, Worcestershire sauce, thyme, salt, and pepper. Mix well.

- Form the mixture into a loaf shape and place on a baking sheet.

- Toss chopped carrots, celery, and red onion with olive oil, salt, and pepper. Arrange the vegetables around the meatloaf on the baking sheet.

- Bake for 50-60 minutes, or until the meatloaf is cooked through and vegetables are tender.

Spiced Lentil Soup with Coconut Milk and Spinach

Ingredients:

- 1 tablespoon olive oil

- 1 onion, chopped

- 2 carrots, chopped

- 2 celery stalks, chopped

- 2 cloves garlic, minced

- 1 teaspoon ground cumin

- 1/2 teaspoon turmeric

- 1/4 teaspoon ground coriander

- 1 (14.5 oz) can diced tomatoes, undrained

- 4 cups vegetable broth

- 1 cup brown lentils, rinsed

- 1 (13.5 oz) can coconut milk (light)

- 2 cups chopped spinach

- Salt and pepper to taste

Instructions:

- Heat olive oil in a large pot over medium heat. Add onion, carrots, and celery, and cook until softened, about 5 minutes.

- Stir in garlic, cumin, turmeric, and coriander. Cook for an additional minute.

- Add diced tomatoes, vegetable broth, lentils, and coconut milk. Bring to a boil, then reduce heat and simmer for 30 minutes, or until lentils are tender.

- Stir in chopped spinach and cook for an additional 2-3 minutes, or until wilted.

- Season with salt and pepper to taste.

Korean BBQ Beef Lettuce Wraps with Kimchi Slaw

Ingredients:

- 1 pound flank steak, thinly sliced

- 1/4 cup soy sauce (low-sodium)

- 1 tablespoon brown sugar

- 1 tablespoon rice vinegar

- 1 tablespoon sesame oil

- 1 clove garlic, minced

- 1 teaspoon grated ginger

- 1/2 teaspoon red pepper flakes (adjust for desired spice level)

For the Kimchi Slaw:

- 1 cup shredded green cabbage

- 1/2 cup chopped kimchi (adjust for desired spice level)

- 1 carrot, julienned

* 2 tablespoons rice vinegar

* 1 tablespoon sesame oil

* 1 teaspoon soy sauce (low-sodium)

For Serving:

* Bibb lettuce leaves

Instructions:

* In a bowl, combine soy sauce, brown sugar, rice vinegar, sesame oil, garlic, ginger, and red pepper flakes. Marinate sliced beef for at least 30 minutes.

* While beef marinates, prepare the kimchi slaw. In a bowl, combine shredded cabbage, chopped kimchi, julienned carrot, rice vinegar, sesame oil, and soy sauce. Toss to combine and chill in the refrigerator.

* Heat a grill pan or skillet over medium-high heat. Cook marinated beef for 1-2 minutes per side, or until desired doneness.

- Serve cooked beef in Bibb lettuce leaves with kimchi slaw on the side.

Mediterranean Chickpea Salad Bowls with Whole Wheat Pita Bread

Ingredients:

- 1 (15 oz) can chickpeas, rinsed and drained

- 1 cucumber, chopped

- 1 tomato, chopped

- 1/2 cup chopped red onion

- 1/4 cup crumbled feta cheese (optional)

- 1/4 cup chopped kalamata olives

- 1 tablespoon olive oil

- 1 tablespoon lemon juice

- 1 teaspoon dried oregano

- Salt and pepper to taste

For Serving:

- Whole wheat pita bread, warmed

Instructions:

- In a bowl, combine chickpeas, cucumber, tomato, red onion, feta cheese (optional), and kalamata olives.

- In a separate bowl, whisk together olive oil, lemon juice, oregano, salt, and pepper.

- Pour the dressing over the chickpea salad and toss to coat.

- Serve chickpea salad bowls with warmed whole wheat pita bread.

Summer Berry and Chia Seed Pudding with Coconut Milk

Ingredients:

- 1 cup mixed berries (fresh or frozen)

- 1/2 cup chia seeds

- 1 1/2 cups coconut milk (full-fat or light)

- 1/4 cup honey or maple syrup (optional)

- 1 teaspoon vanilla extract

- Fresh berries and mint leaves (for garnish, optional)

Instructions:

- In a bowl or jar, combine berries, chia seeds, coconut milk, honey or maple syrup (optional), and vanilla extract. Stir well.

- Cover and refrigerate for at least 4 hours, or overnight, for the chia seeds to absorb the liquid and pudding to thicken.

- When ready to serve, spoon pudding into bowls and garnish with fresh berries and mint leaves (optional).

One-Pan Lemon Garlic Salmon with Roasted Asparagus

Ingredients:

- 2 salmon fillets

- 1 tablespoon olive oil

- Salt and pepper to taste

- 1 lemon, sliced

- 2 cloves garlic, minced

- 1 bunch asparagus, trimmed

Instructions:

- Preheat oven to 400°F (200°C). Season salmon fillets with olive oil, salt, and pepper.

- Place salmon fillets on a baking sheet. Top with lemon slices and sprinkle with minced garlic.

- Toss asparagus with a drizzle of olive oil, salt, and pepper. Arrange asparagus spears around the salmon on the baking sheet.

- Bake for 15-20 minutes, or until salmon is cooked through and asparagus is tender-crisp.

Thai Coconut Curry with Tofu and Vegetables

Ingredients:

- 1 tablespoon olive oil

- 1 onion, chopped

- 2 cloves garlic, minced

- 1 tablespoon red curry paste (adjust for desired spice level)

- 1 (13.5 oz) can coconut milk (light)

- 1 cup vegetable broth

- 1 block (14 oz) firm tofu, drained and cubed

- 1 cup chopped bell pepper (any color)

- 1 cup broccoli florets

- 1/2 cup snow peas

- 1/4 cup chopped fresh cilantro

- Cooked brown rice (for serving)

Instructions:

- Heat olive oil in a large pot or Dutch oven over medium heat. Add onion and cook until softened, about 5 minutes.

- Stir in garlic and red curry paste. Cook for an additional minute, allowing the curry paste to release its fragrance.

- Add coconut milk and vegetable broth. Bring to a simmer.

- Add cubed tofu, bell pepper, broccoli florets, and snow peas. Simmer for 10-15 minutes, or until vegetables are tender-crisp and tofu is heated through.

- Stir in chopped cilantro and adjust seasonings with salt and pepper if desired.

- Serve Thai coconut curry over cooked brown rice.

Mexican Quinoa Bowl with Black Beans and Avocado Crema

Ingredients:

- 1 cup cooked quinoa

- 1 (15 oz) can black beans, rinsed and drained

- 1/2 cup chopped corn (fresh, frozen, or canned)

- 1/4 cup chopped red onion

- 1/4 cup chopped fresh cilantro

- 1/4 cup crumbled queso fresco cheese (optional)

For the Avocado Crema:

- 1/2 avocado, mashed

- 1 tablespoon lime juice

- 1/4 cup chopped fresh cilantro

- Salt and pepper to taste

For Serving:

- Optional toppings: Sliced jalapenos, chopped tomatoes, crumbled tortilla chips

Instructions:

- Prepare cooked quinoa according to package instructions.

- In a bowl, combine cooked quinoa, black beans, corn, red onion, and cilantro.

- To make the avocado crema, mash avocado with lime juice, cilantro, salt, and pepper in a small bowl.

- Assemble bowls with quinoa mixture, top with avocado crema, and sprinkle with queso fresco cheese (optional).

- Offer sliced jalapenos, chopped tomatoes, and crumbled tortilla chips for additional toppings.

Tuna Salad Lettuce Wraps with Asian Slaw

Ingredients:

- 2 (5 oz) cans tuna in water, drained

- 1/4 cup chopped celery

- 1/4 cup chopped red onion

- 2 tablespoons mayonnaise (light or low-fat)

- 1 tablespoon lemon juice

- 1/4 teaspoon dried dill

- Salt and pepper to taste

For the Asian Slaw:

- 2 cups shredded green cabbage

- 1 carrot, julienned

- 1/4 cup chopped red bell pepper

- 2 tablespoons rice vinegar

- 1 tablespoon soy sauce (low-sodium)

- 1 teaspoon sesame oil

For Serving:

- Bibb lettuce leaves or romaine lettuce hearts

Instructions:

- In a bowl, combine flaked tuna, chopped celery, red onion, mayonnaise, lemon juice, dill, salt, and pepper. Mix well.

- To make the Asian slaw, combine shredded cabbage, julienned carrot, chopped red bell pepper, rice vinegar, soy sauce, and sesame oil in a bowl. Toss to combine and chill in the refrigerator for at least 15 minutes.

- Serve tuna salad mixture in Bibb lettuce leaves or romaine lettuce hearts. Top with Asian slaw.

Roasted Brussels Sprouts with Balsamic Glaze and Pecans

Ingredients:

- 1 pound Brussels sprouts, trimmed and halved

- 1 tablespoon olive oil

- Salt and pepper to taste

- 1/4 cup balsamic vinegar

- 1 tablespoon brown sugar

- 1/4 cup chopped pecans, toasted

Instructions:

- Preheat oven to 400°F (200°C). Toss Brussels sprouts with olive oil, salt, and pepper. Spread on a baking sheet in a single layer.

- Roast for 20-25 minutes, or until tender-crisp and slightly browned.

- While Brussels sprouts roast, prepare the glaze. In a small saucepan, combine balsamic vinegar and brown sugar. Heat over medium heat until the sugar dissolves and the mixture thickens slightly, about 5 minutes.

- Toss roasted Brussels sprouts with the balsamic glaze. Top with chopped pecans and serve.

Mediterranean Chickpea Fritters with Lemon Yogurt Sauce

Ingredients:

- 1 (15 oz) can chickpeas, rinsed and drained

- 1/2 cup chopped red onion

- 1/4 cup chopped fresh parsley

- 1/4 cup crumbled feta cheese (optional)

- 1/4 cup chickpea flour (or all-purpose flour)

- 1 egg, beaten

- Salt and pepper to taste

For the Lemon Yogurt Sauce:

- 1/2 cup plain Greek yogurt (2% or non-fat)

- 1 tablespoon lemon juice

- 1 tablespoon olive oil

- 1/4 teaspoon dried dill

- Salt and pepper to taste

Instructions:

- In a food processor, pulse together chickpeas, red onion, parsley, feta cheese (optional), chickpea flour, and egg until a coarse mixture forms. Season with salt and pepper.

- Heat a thin layer of olive oil in a skillet over medium heat. Scoop the chickpea mixture by tablespoons and flatten slightly into patties.

- Cook for 3-4 minutes per side, or until golden brown and crispy.

- To make the lemon yogurt sauce, whisk together Greek yogurt, lemon juice, olive oil, dill, salt, and pepper in a small bowl.

- Serve chickpea fritters with lemon yogurt sauce on the side.

Coconut Curry Cauliflower Rice with Shrimp

Ingredients:

- 1 head of cauliflower, riced

- 1 tablespoon olive oil

- 1 onion, chopped

- 2 cloves garlic, minced

- 1 tablespoon red curry paste (adjust for desired spice level)

- 1 (13.5 oz) can coconut milk (light)

- 1 cup vegetable broth

- 1 pound shrimp, peeled and deveined

- 1/2 cup chopped green beans

- 1/4 cup chopped fresh cilantro

- Lime wedges (for serving)

Instructions:

- Heat olive oil in a large pot or Dutch oven over medium heat. Add onion and cook until softened, about 5 minutes.

- Stir in garlic and red curry paste. Cook for an additional minute, allowing the curry paste to release its fragrance.

- Add coconut milk and vegetable broth. Bring to a simmer.

- Add cauliflower rice and simmer for 10 minutes, or until tender-crisp.

- In the last few minutes of cooking, add shrimp and green beans. Cook until shrimp are pink and cooked through, about 3-5 minutes.

- Stir in chopped cilantro and adjust seasonings with salt and pepper if desired.

- Serve coconut curry cauliflower rice with shrimp and lime wedges for squeezing.

Turkey Meatloaf Muffins with Roasted Vegetables

Ingredients:

- 1 pound ground turkey

- 1/2 cup chopped onion

- 1/4 cup chopped bell pepper (any color)

- 1/4 cup chopped mushrooms

- 1/4 cup rolled oats

- 1 egg, beaten

- 1 tablespoon Worcestershire sauce

- 1 teaspoon dried thyme

- Salt and pepper to taste

For the Roasted Vegetables:

- 2 medium carrots, chopped

- 2 celery stalks, chopped

- 1 red onion, chopped

- 1 tablespoon olive oil

- Salt and pepper to taste

Instructions:

- Preheat oven to 375°F (190°C). In a large bowl, combine ground turkey, onion, bell pepper, mushrooms, rolled oats, egg, Worcestershire sauce, thyme, salt, and pepper. Mix well.

- Divide the mixture into muffin tins lined with paper liners.

- Toss chopped carrots, celery, and red onion with olive oil, salt, and pepper. Arrange the vegetables around the meatloaf muffins on the baking sheet.

- Bake for 30-35 minutes, or until the meatloaf muffins are cooked through and vegetables are tender.

Summer Berry Smoothie Bowl with Chia Seeds and Granola

Ingredients:

- 1 cup frozen mixed berries

- 1/2 cup unsweetened almond milk (or other plant-based milk)

- 1/4 cup chopped banana

- 1 tablespoon chia seeds

- 1/4 cup granola (low-sugar or homemade)

- Fresh berries and mint leaves (for garnish, optional)

Instructions:

- In a blender, combine frozen berries, almond milk, banana, and chia seeds. Blend until smooth and creamy.

- Pour the smoothie into a bowl and top with granola, fresh berries, and mint leaves (optional).

THANKS   FOR

READING

THIS BOOK.